PRETERM BABY

A guide to understanding and preventing the leading cause of preterm birth

JAMES BIRKHOFF

All rights reserved. No part of this publication may be reproduced, distributed or transmitted in any form or by any means, including photocopying, recording or other electronic or mechanical methods, without the prior written permission of the publisher, except in the case of brief quotations embodied in critical reviews and certain other non-commercial uses permitted by copyright law.

Copyright © James Birkhoff, 2023

TABLE OF CONTENT

CHAPTER 1
CHAPTER 2
CHAPTER 3
CHAPTER 4
CHAPTER 5
CHAPTER 6
CHAPTER 7

INTRODUCTION

One in ten newborns worldwide suffers from preterm birth, a serious health problem. It takes place when a baby is born before the 37th week of pregnancy, when the pregnancy is considered to be full-term. A baby's health can be seriously affected by a preterm birth, which can cause problems with breathing, feeding, and an increased risk of infections. It may also result in developmental delays and long-term health issues in some instances, such as an increased risk for chronic health conditions such as asthma and diabetes. There are several factors that can increase the risk of preterm birth, including certain medical conditions in the mother, such as high blood pressure or diabetes, as well as lifestyle factors such as smoking or substance abuse. Some women may be at higher risk due to a previous history of preterm birth or other pregnancy complications.

Prevention of preterm birth is an important area of research, as even a small reduction in the rate of preterm birth can have a significant impact on the health of newborns and the overall population. Treatment for preterm babies often involves specialized care in a neonatal intensive care unit (NICU), where medical professionals can provide the necessary support and treatment for the baby to survive and thrive.

There are several categories of preterm birth:

- Late preterm birth: This refers to birth between 34 and 36 weeks of pregnancy. Babies born at this gestational age are at an increased risk of health problems, but they generally have a better prognosis than babies born earlier.

- Moderately preterm birth: This refers to birth between 32 and 34 weeks of pregnancy. Babies born at this gestational age are at a higher risk of health problems than those born later, but they generally have a better prognosis than babies born earlier.

- Very preterm birth: This refers to birth before 32 weeks of pregnancy. Babies born at this gestational age are at a very high risk of health problems and may require specialized care in a neonatal intensive care unit (NICU).

- Extremely preterm birth: This refers to birth before 28 weeks of pregnancy. Babies born at this gestational age are at a very high risk of health problems and may require a great deal of medical intervention in order to survive.

It is impossible to overstate the significance of comprehending preterm birth. Preterm birth has a significant impact on families, healthcare systems, and society as a whole, and it is a leading cause of infant death and disability. However, many preterm infants can live healthy lives with the right medical care. Preterm birth's causes, risk factors, symptoms and signs, diagnosis, treatment options, prevention, and coping strategies are all covered in detail in this guide. Families will gain a better understanding of the difficulties associated with preterm birth and the steps they can take to ensure their baby has the best possible outcome thanks to the information in this guide. This guide can also be used by healthcare professionals to educate families and give them the support they need during this trying time.

Preterm birth is a complicated problem whose causes and best ways to avoid it are still poorly understood. However, families, medical professionals, and researchers can collaborate to improve outcomes for babies and families affected by preterm birth and reduce the incidence of the condition.

CHAPTER 1
Definition and types of preterm birth

Preterm birth, also known as premature birth, is defined as the birth of a baby before 37 weeks of pregnancy. Preterm birth can have serious health consequences for the newborn, as the earlier a baby is born, the greater the risk of complications.

There are two main types of preterm birth: spontaneous and induced.

1. Spontaneous preterm birth is the type of preterm birth that occurs when labor begins on its own, before the pregnancy has reached full term (37 weeks). There are several potential causes of spontaneous preterm birth, including:

- Premature rupture of the membranes (the water breaks before labor starts)

- Uterine contractions that cause the cervix to open

- Separation of the placenta from the uterine wall

There are a number of factors that can increase the risk of spontaneous preterm birth, including:

- Previous preterm birth: Women who have had a preterm birth before are at higher risk of having another preterm birth.

- Short cervix: A cervix that measures less than 25 millimeters (mm) in length is more likely to open prematurely.

- Infection: Certain infections, such as sexually transmitted infections (STIs), urinary tract infections (UTIs), and vaginal infections, can increase the risk of preterm birth.

- Medical conditions: Certain medical conditions, such as high blood pressure, diabetes, and autoimmune disorders, can increase the risk of preterm birth.

- Environmental factors: Exposure to certain environmental toxins, such as tobacco smoke, can increase the risk of preterm birth.

It is important to try to prevent spontaneous preterm birth whenever possible, as it can have serious consequences for both the mother and the baby. However, in some cases, it may not be possible to prevent spontaneous preterm birth, and the focus will be on managing the delivery and providing the best possible care for the mother and the baby.

2. Induced preterm birth is the deliberate delivery of a baby before it has reached full term, which is typically around 37-41 weeks of pregnancy. This can be done medically, through the use of drugs or other medical procedures, or surgically, through a cesarean delivery or induction of labor.

There are a number of reasons why a healthcare provider may recommend inducing preterm labor, including:

- The mother has a medical condition that poses a risk to her or the baby's health, such as pre-eclampsia or gestational diabetes

- The baby is not growing properly or has stopped growing in the womb

- The mother's water has broken, but labor has not started

- The placenta is not functioning properly

- The mother is carrying multiples (twins, triplets, etc.) and one or more of the babies is not getting enough nutrients and oxygen

Induced preterm birth can carry some risks, including:

- The baby may not be fully developed and may be at an increased risk of health problems or complications

- The mother may experience complications during labor and delivery, such as bleeding or infection

- The baby may have difficulty breastfeeding or establishing a strong bond with the mother

It is important for expectant mothers to discuss the potential risks and benefits of induced preterm birth with their healthcare provider, and to consider all options carefully before making a decision.

CHAPTER 2
Causes and risk factors of preterm birth

Preterm birth is a major public health problem and a major cause of infant mortality and morbidity. Preterm birth can be caused by a variety of factors, many of which are unknown. The following are some of the known causes of preterm birth:

- Premature birth: The uterus begins to contract and the cervix begins to open before 37 weeks of pregnancy, which is the most common cause of preterm birth.

- Problems with the placenta: Preterm birth can be caused by abnormalities in the placenta, such as placental abruption (where the placenta separates from the uterine wall before birth) or placental insufficiency (where the placenta does not provide the baby with enough oxygen and nutrients).

- Infections: The risk of having a baby before the due date can be heightened by certain infections, such as those transmitted sexually and infections of the urinary tract.

- Praevia placenta: The placenta may cover all or part of the cervix—the neck of the womb—at times when it attaches low down in the uterus. The placenta usually moves up and out of the way as the pregnancy goes on, but sometimes it doesn't. If the placenta is less than 20 millimeters from the cervix, it is referred to as low-lying placenta, while if it covers the cervix, it is referred to as placenta praevia. You are more likely to give birth early if you have placenta praevia.

- Pregnancies with more than one child: Premature births of twins and triplets are frequent. Most triplets and more than half of twins are born before 37 weeks. Even if you don't go into labor too early, you might be told to give birth before your due date to avoid complications. Women who are expecting multiple children do not typically receive progesterone pessaries, cervical stitches, or the Arabin Pessary—all of which have the potential to prevent premature birth. Additionally, bed rest is rarely recommended. During your pregnancy, you may be prescribed corticosteroids to speed up your baby's lungs' development. Premature birth-related complications may be less likely as a result of this.

- Low levels of PAPP-A: The hormone known as Pregnancy Associated Plasma Protein-A (PAPP-A) is produced by the placenta during pregnancy. It is measured as part of the prenatal screenings you get before you get pregnant. The placenta, the organ that helps the baby grow and develop, may not function as well if there are low levels of PAPP-A. Preeclampsia or premature birth may occur more frequently. If you are found to have low levels of PAPP-A, you will probably be given more scans to watch your baby grow. Additionally, it is essential to become familiar with your baby's movements and to immediately notify your midwife or maternity unit if you believe your baby's movements have slowed down, stopped, or changed. Learn more about keeping an eye on your baby's movements. Your midwife will also tell you not to smoke because it can slow down your baby's growth and affect how your placenta works.

- Syndrome of antiphospholipids (APS): An immune system blood disorder known as antiphospholipid syndrome can result in complications during pregnancy, including a premature birth. You might be able to be referred for tests to try to figure out why you've had repeated or late miscarriages. This might include APS tests. Treatment can increase your chances of getting pregnant successfully if you are diagnosed. Throughout your pregnancy, you will also be closely monitored. The best thing you can do if you already know you have APS is talk to your general practitioner or specialist before getting pregnant, or as soon as possible if you are already pregnant. This is due to the fact that the treatment you need to increase your chances of having a healthy pregnancy is most effective when started as soon as possible.

- Choices you make in your life that can increase your risk of having a baby too soon: There is clear evidence that your lifestyle can affect your pregnancy, so you can try to reduce your risk of having a baby too soon.

- Addiction to alcohol: During pregnancy, excessive alcohol consumption raises the risk of premature birth as well as; low birth weight, learning difficulties, and behavioral issues for the baby in later life. Alcohol enters your baby through the placenta and your blood when you drink. Since there is no known safe level of alcohol consumption during pregnancy, the safest course of action is not to drink at all.

- Premature birth and smoking: The most preventable factor in problems and loss during pregnancy is smoking. Additionally, it raises the risk of preterm birth and; ectopic pregnancy, stillbirth, sudden infant death syndrome, and miscarriage. To quit smoking, you can do so at any time. Keeping a smoke-free pregnancy helps your baby's health and development.

- Polyhydramnios, or an excess of amniotic fluid, is: The fluid that surrounds your infant during pregnancy is called amniotic fluid. During pregnancy, polyhydramnios occurs when there is excessive amniotic fluid surrounding the baby. This slightly raises the risk of complications during pregnancy, including a premature birth. During pregnancy, excessive fluid buildup can be caused by a variety of factors, including but not limited to: diabetes and gestational diabetes, multiple pregnancies, an infection during pregnancy, a blockage in the baby's gut (gut atresia), the baby's blood cells being attacked by the mother's blood cells (rhesus disease), or your baby having a genetic condition During a checkup in the latter stages of pregnancy, excessive amniotic fluid is typically detected. It usually doesn't mean anything serious, but you'll probably get more checks while you're pregnant. However, try not to be concerned because most babies born to mothers with polyhydramnios will be healthy. If you have any questions or concerns, talk to your midwife or doctor.

- Prior prematurity birth: Women who have previously had a preterm birth are more likely to have another one.

- Abnormalities of the uterus (womb with unusual shape): A uterus that formed in an unusual manner prior to birth is known as a uterine abnormality. There may be a greater chance of preterm birth depending on the shape of the womb. When they become pregnant, the majority of women are unaware that they may have an abnormally shaped uterus. Investigations for infertility or miscarriage typically uncover it.

- Short time between conceptions: Preterm birth is more common in women who conceive again within a short time after giving birth.

- Pre-eclampsia: A condition known as pre-eclampsia affects some pregnant women. Proteinuria and high blood pressure, also known as hypertension, are the two symptoms. Pre-eclampsia typically appears after the 20th week of pregnancy or shortly after the birth of the baby. Pre-eclampsia symptoms can be mild or severe. Pregnancy early may be recommended if severe pre-eclampsia is present.

- After 24 weeks, bleeding: After the first trimester, bleeding may indicate a problem with the placenta, such as a placental abruption or a low-lying placenta, both of which can lead to preterm birth. Even if you don't have any other symptoms, any bleeding during pregnancy should be looked into. If you are bleeding when you are more than 12 weeks pregnant, go to your local A&E or call the hospital's maternity unit right away to get checked just in case.

- Transfusion syndrome involving twins (TTTS): The same blood supply is shared by monochorionic pregnancies—twins with a common placenta—as well. Uneven blood flow may occur in approximately 15 out of every 100 monochorionic twin pregnancies. This indicates that one baby receives insufficient blood and experiences low blood pressure, while the other baby receives insufficient blood and experiences high blood pressure. Twin-to-twin transfusion syndrome (TTTS) refers to this condition. Premature birth is sometimes the result of TTTS. You will be checked for signs of TTTS with frequent scans if you are carrying twins.

- Diabetes types 1 and 2: One of the most prevalent issues associated with diabetes and pregnancy is premature birth. However, taking good care of your blood sugar levels before and during pregnancy will help lower the risk.

- Early water breaking (PPROM): When your waters break before labour begins before 37 weeks of pregnancy, you have preterm prelabour rupture of membranes (PPROM).

Within the first week after their waters break, approximately half of women with PPROM will go into labour. The likelihood of going into labour within one week of your water breaking increases with the pregnancy stage. Three to four out of every ten premature births are linked to PPROM. You should get in touch with your doctor as soon as possible and go to the hospital for a checkup if you think your waters may have broken.

- Diabetes at birth: If the healthcare team is concerned about the health of the mother or the baby and the likelihood of complications, it may be recommended to women with gestational diabetes to have an early delivery via induction or caesarean section. Additionally, some studies have demonstrated that pregnant women with gestational diabetes are more likely to give birth prematurely. Try not to worry, though. When gestational diabetes is properly diagnosed and managed during pregnancy, most women have healthy pregnancies and healthy babies.

- Social or psychological stress: Premature birth is linked to severe stress or depression during pregnancy, according to some research, but why? This stress may frequently be accompanied by related issues like a lack of social support, emotional abuse, or domestic violence, as well as behaviors that some people engage in when they are experiencing severe stress, such as poor eating habits or smoking. When you are pregnant, it is normal to experience some levels of stress or anxiety. However, you may require assistance if you are experiencing these feelings. It can be difficult to tell whether your feelings are manageable or a sign of something more serious during pregnancy, which can be a very emotional time. Have self-assurance. You can tell if your feelings are normal for you the best. There are no standards about how pushed you should be prior to conversing with your birthing specialist how you feel. If you have any concerns while you are pregnant, you can talk to a doctor or other medical professional at any time. If you need assistance, you can get it sooner if you ask for it sooner.

- Issues with your cervix, including a weak cervix: During pregnancy, the womb's neck, or cervix, may sometimes shorten, which may indicate preterm birth. The reason for this may or may not be known by doctors, but it can occur if the cervix has been damaged. For instance, as a result of a tear that occurs during childbirth or as part of treatment for an abnormal cervical screening, such as a largo loop excision of the transformation zone (LLETZ) or a cone biopsy. The cervix is referred to as weak or incompetent when this occurs, indicating that it may open or shorten earlier. This could result in a premature birth. You may be offered a cervical stitch, also known as a cerclage or cervical suture, or hormone treatment, such as progesterone, to prevent your baby from being born prematurely if scans reveal a problem with your cervix.

- Restrictions on foetal growth (FGR): A condition known as foetal growth restriction (FGR) occurs when a baby grows slower or stops growing during pregnancy or is smaller than expected. Intrauterine growth restriction (IUGR) is another name for it. There is a greater chance of complications during pregnancy if your baby has FGR. The baby's development and health will be closely monitored by your healthcare team, and you may be advised to give birth earlier than your due date.

- Weight: Premature birth is more common in women who are either overweight or underweight when they become pregnant. Your midwife may take measurements of your height and weight to determine your body mass index (BMI) during your first antenatal visit, also known as the booking appointment. Using your height and weight, you can determine if your weight is healthy using your BMI. If someone working with your health care uses the terms "underweight," "overweight," or "obese" to describe your weight, try not to be offended. These terms are not liked by many women, but no one is judging you. They might have to be used by the doctors who are taking care of you during your pregnancy so that they can make sure you get the best advice and support to help you have a healthy pregnancy.

- Lack of nutrition: Premature birth may be more likely if a pregnant woman receives insufficient nutrition.

It is essential to note that the cause of preterm birth is frequently unknown. Prenatal care should be provided on a regular basis to expectant mothers in order to identify and address any problems that may arise.

CHAPTER 3

Diagnosis and screening for preterm birth

A premature birth can have serious effects on the baby's health, such as an increased risk of respiratory issues, difficulties with feeding, and developmental delays.

A healthcare professional typically bases a diagnosis of preterm birth on the length of the pregnancy and the presence of labor signs. The cervix, which is the lower part of the uterus that opens during childbirth, may be measured by the provider to determine whether it is dilated or effaced. They might also check for contractions, which are strong, regular muscle contractions that help push the baby out of the womb during labor.

Preterm birth can also be diagnosed using other diagnostic procedures like:

- Ultrasound: An ultrasound is a non-invasive procedure that shows the baby and the uterus through high-frequency sound waves. An ultrasound can help the doctor figure out how big the baby is, how old it is, and look for any problems.

- Test for fetal fibronectin: A sample of the discharge from the cervix and vagina is taken for this test to see if fetal fibronectin, a protein, is present. Amniotic fluid test: The presence of this protein may indicate that the woman is at risk for preterm birth. The amount of amniotic fluid, which surrounds and protects the baby in the uterus, is measured during this test. A sign of preterm labor can be a low level of amniotic fluid.

- Monitor for contractures: The strength and frequency of contractions can be measured with a monitor. This may assist in determining whether the woman is having an early delivery.

- Profile biophysique (BPP): The non-stress test in this procedure, which measures the fetal heart rate in response to movement, is combined with an ultrasound. A higher risk of preterm birth may be indicated by a low BPP score.

- Exam of the pelvis: Your healthcare provider may conduct a pelvic exam as part of a routine prenatal visit to check for any changes, such as cervical dilation or effacement (thinning of the cervix), that could indicate an increased risk of preterm labor.

The healthcare provider will work with the expectant mother to try to delay delivery for as long as possible to give the baby more time to grow and develop if there is a possibility of preterm birth. Bed rest, medications to stop the contractions, or other treatments may be necessary.

CHAPTER 4

Complications of preterm birth for the infant

Although not all premature infants experience complications, premature birth can result in short- and long-term health issues. In general, complications are more likely to occur when a baby is born earlier. Additionally, birth weight is a significant factor. While some issues may manifest at birth, others may not until later.

COMPLICATIONS IN THE SHORT TERM

In the first few weeks, the following problems may arise from a premature birth:

- Breathing difficulties: Due to an immature respiratory system, a premature infant may experience breathing difficulties. Because the lungs are unable to expand and contract normally, the baby may develop respiratory distress syndrome if the lungs lack surfactant, a substance that allows the lungs to expand. Bronchopulmonary dysplasia is another lung disorder that can occur in premature infants. Additionally, breathing pauses known as apnea may occur in some premature babies.

- Heart issues: Low blood pressure (hypotension) and patent ductus arteriosus (PDA) are the most common heart conditions in premature infants. An ongoing gap exists between the pulmonary artery and the aorta in the PDA. Although this defect typically heals on its own, if left untreated, it can result in heart failure, a heart murmur, and other complications. Medications, intravenous fluid adjustments, and occasionally blood transfusions may be required for low blood pressure.

- Problems with the brain: There is a greater chance of an intraventricular hemorrhage—brain bleeding—the earlier a baby is born. The majority of hemorrhages are mild and disappear quickly. However, larger brain bleeding in some infants may result in permanent brain damage.

- Issues with temperature control: Infants born prematurely can rapidly lose body heat. They are unable to generate sufficient heat to compensate for what is lost through their bodies' surface because they lack the stored body fat of full-term infants. An abnormally low core body temperature (hypothermia) can occur when the body temperature drops too low. Premature infants who are hypothermic may experience difficulties breathing and low blood sugar levels. Premature infants may also expend all of their energy from feedings just to keep warm. Because of this, small premature babies need more heat from a warmer or an incubator until they grow up and can keep their body temperature on their own.

- Problems with the digestive system: Necrotizing enterocolitis (NEC) is a complication that can occur in premature infants who have immature gastrointestinal systems. Premature infants who begin to eat can develop this potentially fatal condition in which damaged cells line the bowel wall. Breastfed premature infants have a significantly lower risk of developing NEC.

- Blood issues: Anaemia and newborn jaundice are two blood conditions that can affect premature infants. Anaemia is a common condition in which there are insufficient red blood cells in the body. During the first few months of life, all newborns experience a gradual decrease in their red blood cell count; however, this decrease may be more pronounced in premature infants. A yellow discoloration in a newborn's eyes and skin is known as newborn jaundice. This condition is caused by an excess of the yellow-coloured substance bilirubin, which comes from the liver or red blood cells. There are numerous causes of jaundice, but preterm babies are more likely to develop it.

- Problems with metabolism: Metabolism issues are common in premature infants. Hypoglycemia, an abnormally low level of glucose in the blood, can occur in some premature babies. Premature infants typically have smaller glucose stores than full-term infants, so this may occur. Additionally, it is more challenging for premature babies to convert their stored glucose into active, more usable forms.

- Issues with the immune system: Premature babies frequently have a weaker immune system, which can increase the likelihood of infection. Premature infant infections can quickly spread to the bloodstream, resulting in sepsis, a bloodstream infection.

COMPLICATIONS IN THE LONG TERM

In the long term, premature birth may result in the following problems:

- Palsy of the head: A disorder of movement, muscle tone, or posture known as cerebral palsy can be brought on by an infection, insufficient blood flow, or injury to the developing brain of a newborn either early in pregnancy or while the baby is still young and immature. Impairment in learning On various developmental milestones, premature babies are more likely to lag behind full-term counterparts. A child who was born prematurely may be more likely to have learning disabilities when they reach school age.

- Vision issues: Retinopathy of prematurity is a condition in which the light-sensitive nerve layer at the back of the eye (retina) experiences swelling and overgrowth of blood vessels. Premature infants may develop this condition. The abnormal retinal vessels may occasionally pull the retina out of place by gradually scarring it. Retinal detachment is a condition that, if left untreated, has the potential to impair vision and result in blindness. It occurs when the retina is pulled away from the back of the eye.

- Issues with hearing: Hearing loss in some form is more common in premature infants. Before going home, all babies will have their hearing checked.

- Dental issues: Dental issues like tooth discoloration, improperly aligned teeth, and delayed tooth eruption are more common in critically ill premature infants.

- Problems with one's mental and physical health: Premature infants may be more likely than full-term infants to have developmental delays and certain behavioural or psychological issues.

- Issues with chronic health: When compared to full-term infants, premature infants are more likely to have chronic health issues, some of which may necessitate hospitalisation. Asthma, infections, and feeding issues are more likely to arise or persist. SIDS (sudden infant death syndrome) is also more common in premature infants.

It's important to remember that not all preterm babies will experience these problems. However, it is essential for parents of preterm children to be aware of the potential dangers and to collaborate closely with their child's doctor to ensure that their child receives the appropriate medical attention and support.

CHAPTER 5
Management and treatment of preterm birth

Preterm birth is a common pregnancy complication that can result in serious health issues for the baby. Preterm birth management is determined by the baby's gestational age and the particulars of the pregnancy. Preterm birth can be managed and the baby's outcomes improved using a variety of methods. These are some:

- Corticosteroids during pregnancy: These medications can be administered to the mother prior to delivery to assist in the maturation of the baby's lungs and lower the likelihood of respiratory issues.

- Medication for tocolytics: Preterm labour can be stopped or slowed down with these medications. They delay delivery for a brief period of time by relaxing the muscles in the uterus.

- Taking progesterone supplements: In some instances, it has been demonstrated that taking progesterone supplements, which are made by the ovaries and reduce the risk of preterm birth.

- Antibiotics: Antibiotics may be administered to the mother if she is at risk for infection to aid in the prevention or treatment of any infections that may arise.

- Close surveillance: Both the mother and the baby will be closely watched to make sure they are healthy and happy. Regular checkups, foetal heart rate monitoring, and any other necessary tests and evaluations could all be part of this.

- Restricted physical activity and bed rest: Pregnant women with a high risk of preterm birth may be advised by doctors to limit their physical activity and stay in bed in order to lower their risk of preterm labour.

- Delivery: In some instances, giving birth as soon as possible may be the best option. Depending on the specifics, this can be accomplished via c-section or vaginal delivery.

- Neonatal intensive care unit (NICU) treatment: A NICU may be required for the baby's specialised care if he or she is born very prematurely or has health issues. The infant might receive nutrition and fluids through an IV or feeding tube, be placed on a ventilator to assist with breathing, and receive any other necessary medical care.

- Care aftercare: Preterm infants are more likely to develop certain health issues and may require ongoing medical care to ensure their optimal health and development.

When developing a plan of care that is appropriate for the particular requirements of the mother and the infant, it is essential to collaborate closely with a healthcare team that includes physicians, nurses, and other specialists.

CHAPTER 6
Prevention and care of preterm birth

Premature birth can be prevented in a variety of ways:

- Receiving regular and early prenatal care: As soon as you suspect you are pregnant, it is essential to begin receiving prenatal care. Your healthcare provider can help you identify any potential issues early on, allowing for prompt treatment.

- Taking care of chronic illnesses: Diabetes and high blood pressure are two chronic conditions that can raise the risk of preterm birth. The risk can be reduced by collaborating with a healthcare professional to manage these conditions.

- Maintaining a healthy diet throughout your pregnancy: Eat a lot of vegetables, fruits, lean proteins, and whole grains. Folic acid and calcium supplements should also be taken.

- Avoiding illegal drugs, alcohol, and tobacco: The risk of preterm birth and other complications may be increased by these substances. Preterm birth can be caused by chronic stress. Exercise, meditation, and speaking with a mental health professional are all important ways to manage stress.

- Keeping certain infections at bay: Infections of the genital tract, for example, have been linked to an increased risk of preterm birth. To cut down on the chance of getting sick, it's critical to have safe sex and to wash one's hands frequently.

- Dietary guidelines: Getting enough folic acid and eating a healthy diet before and during pregnancy can help lower the risk of having a baby before the due date.

- Avoiding the following: During pregnancy, you should stay away from activities that could put too much stress on your body, like lifting heavy objects or playing contact sports.

- Getting treatment with progesterone: Progesterone treatment may be suggested to help lower the risk for women who have a history of preterm birth or are at high risk for preterm birth.

- Utilizing a cervical splint: A cervical cerclage, a surgical procedure that involves sewing the cervix shut to help prevent preterm birth, may be suggested by a healthcare provider in some instances. Typically, only women with a weak cervix or a history of preterm birth are recommended for this.

It is essential to discuss the measures you can take to assist in preventing preterm birth with your healthcare provider. They can offer you advice that is tailored to your particular circumstances.

Coping with the emotional impact of preterm birth

Preterm birth can have a significant emotional impact on both the parents and the child. It is normal to experience a variety of feelings during this difficult and stressful time, such as fear, anxiety, sadness, and guilt. Some ways to deal with the emotional impact of a preterm birth include the following:

- Talk to a trusted person: A trusted friend, family member, or therapist can assist you in processing your feelings and provide you with support.

- Get professional assistance: You should think about getting help from a mental health professional if you are having trouble coping with the emotional effects of a preterm birth. They can support you and help you develop coping mechanisms during this trying time. Take care of your physical health: Improve your overall well-being by taking care of your physical health. This could mean getting enough sleep, eating well, and working out frequently.

- Make time for yourself: Spend some time doing things you enjoy and that help you relax, like reading, taking a bath, or going for a walk.

- Stay up to date: You can feel more in control and less anxious if you are aware of your child's medical care and treatment. Find trustworthy information and ask questions to your healthcare team.

- Set attainable goals: Be honest with yourself about what you can and cannot accomplish and give yourself permission to take things one day at a time are important.

- Seek assistance: Families of preterm babies can get emotional and practical support from a variety of support groups.

Keep in mind that experiencing a variety of emotions following a preterm birth is normal and that you should give yourself time to adjust. Don't be afraid to ask for help if you're having trouble coping.

Taking care of a preterm baby

Although taking care of a preterm baby can be difficult, it can also be a time of great love and bonding. The neonatal intensive care unit (NICU) may be necessary for these infants, who frequently have unique medical requirements. Preterm babies' parents must collaborate closely with the medical team to ensure that their children receive the best possible care. Parents can assist in the care of a preterm baby in a number of ways, including:

- Warm the infant: Preterm infants may have difficulty maintaining their body temperature and have less fat in their bodies. Using a heating pad or blanket to keep the baby warm is essential.

- Feed the infant often: Babies born before their due date may have difficulty eating and need to be fed through a tube or a bottle. Because babies have small stomachs and need to eat frequently, it's important to feed them often.

- Be patient: Preterm infants may require gentle handling because they may be more fragile than full-term infants. When picking up or holding the baby, try to be as gentle as possible and avoid rough handling.

- Follow the advice of the doctor: It is essential to adhere to the preterm baby's care plan and instructions from the doctor. This might entail administering medication to the infant or providing special care for certain conditions.

- Give yourself a break: Premature birth can be physically and emotionally draining to care for. To get you through this trying time, it's important to take care of yourself and get support from loved ones.

- Keeping an eye on your vitals: It is essential to regularly monitor the temperature, heart rate, and breathing of preterm infants because they may be more susceptible to infection and other complications.

- Supporting the respiratory system: Some preterm babies might have trouble breathing, and they might need oxygen therapy or other kinds of support for their breathing.

- Promoting attachment and bonding: Skin-to-skin contact with their parents and frequent cuddling and holding can help preterm infants develop attachment and bonding.

- Establish a quiet and peaceful setting: Because preterm babies are susceptible to being easily stimulated, it is essential to provide them with a calm and quiet environment. Try to limit the number of visitors to the hospital room, dim the lights, and make as little noise as possible.

- Seek assistance: When caring for a preterm infant, it is completely normal to experience feelings of anxiety and overwhelm. It is essential to seek assistance from friends, family, and your healthcare team. You might also want to think about joining a group that helps parents of preterm babies.

- Keep in touch with your baby: You can keep in touch with your baby even if they are in the neonatal intensive care unit (NICU). Hold them as much as you can, read to them, and talk to them. This can benefit your baby's development and help you feel more connected to them.

- Keeping your optimism: Although caring for a preterm infant can be challenging, it is essential for parents to maintain a positive outlook and concentrate on the baby's growth and development. Maintaining a positive outlook, setting goals and milestones, and recognizing small victories are all examples of this. Parents may find that this helps keep them motivated and focused on giving their baby the best care possible.

I hope you find these hints useful. It's always best to talk to a doctor or nurse if you have any specific questions or concerns about taking care of your preterm baby.

CHAPTER 7

Future research and potential therapies for preterm birth

As the leading cause of infant death and disability worldwide, preterm birth is a significant public health issue. Preterm birth is the leading cause of death among children under the age of five, and the World Health Organization (WHO) estimates that approximately 15 million babies are born before their due dates each year. An active field of study is the investigation of the causes of preterm birth and potential treatments for preventing it. Therapies for preventing preterm birth and improving the outcomes of preterm babies are the subject of ongoing research. Some examples of areas of investigation and potential treatments are as follows:

- Identifying factors that could lead to a preterm birth: Genetics, exposures to the environment, and certain medical conditions are just a few of the factors that are being studied by researchers as potential contributors to the increased risk of preterm birth. With this information, it may be possible to target interventions and identify pregnant women at high risk for preterm birth.

- Creating new pharmaceutical treatments: The use of medications to lower the risk of preterm birth is the subject of research at the moment. Progesterone supplements, for instance, have been shown to be effective in some instances, and research into other potential treatments, such as calcium channel blockers and non-steroidal anti-inflammatory drugs (NSAIDs), is ongoing.

- Trying to figure out how to use mechanical cervical barriers: As a means of supporting the cervix and lowering the likelihood of preterm birth, mechanical barriers like cerclage or cervical pessaries—a procedure in which the cervix is closed with suture material—are currently the subject of research.

- Investigating the microbiome's function: Preterm birth may be related to the microbiome, the body's collection of microorganisms. Probiotics and other interventions have the potential to alter the microbiome and lower the risk of preterm birth, according to research on the microbiome and preterm birth.

- Enhancing newborn care: The use of specialized incubators and other technologies to support the baby's development and lower the risk of complications are also being investigated by researchers in an effort to improve the treatment of premature babies.

In general, despite the fact that much progress has been made in comprehending and dealing with preterm birth, there is still a great deal of work to be done to fully comprehend the causes of this complicated condition and to develop efficient therapies for both its prevention and treatment

www.ingramcontent.com/pod-product-compliance
Lightning Source LLC
Chambersburg PA
CBHW071148240526
45465CB00024BA/2093